Sensei Self Development

Mental Health Chronicles Series

*Identifying Your Values
and Priorities*

Sensei Paul David

Copyright Page

Sensei Self Development -
Identifying Your Values and Priorities,
by Sensei Paul David

Copyright © 2024

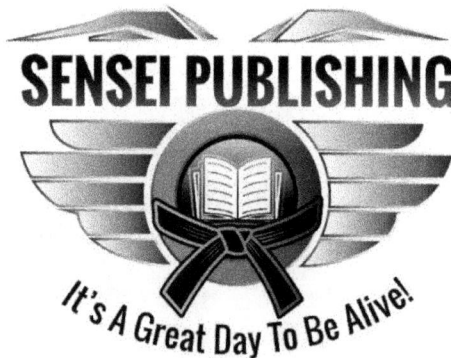

SENSEI PUBLISHING

It's A Great Day To Be Alive!

www.senseipublishing.com

@senseipublishing
#senseipublishing

Get/Share Your FREE SSD Mental Health Chronicles at www.senseiselfdevelopment.care

or

CLICK HERE

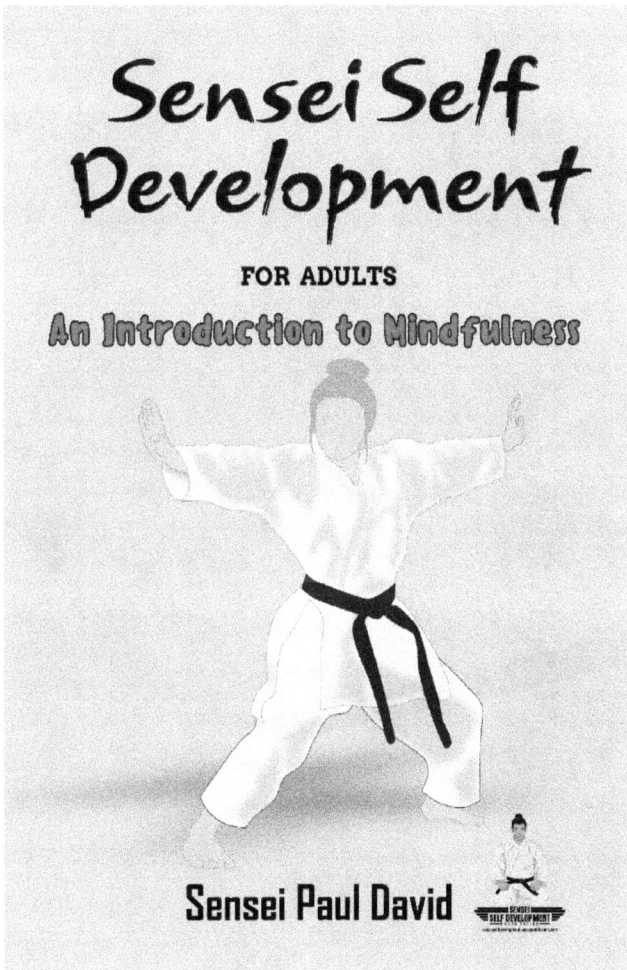

Check Out The SSD Chronicles Series CLICK HERE

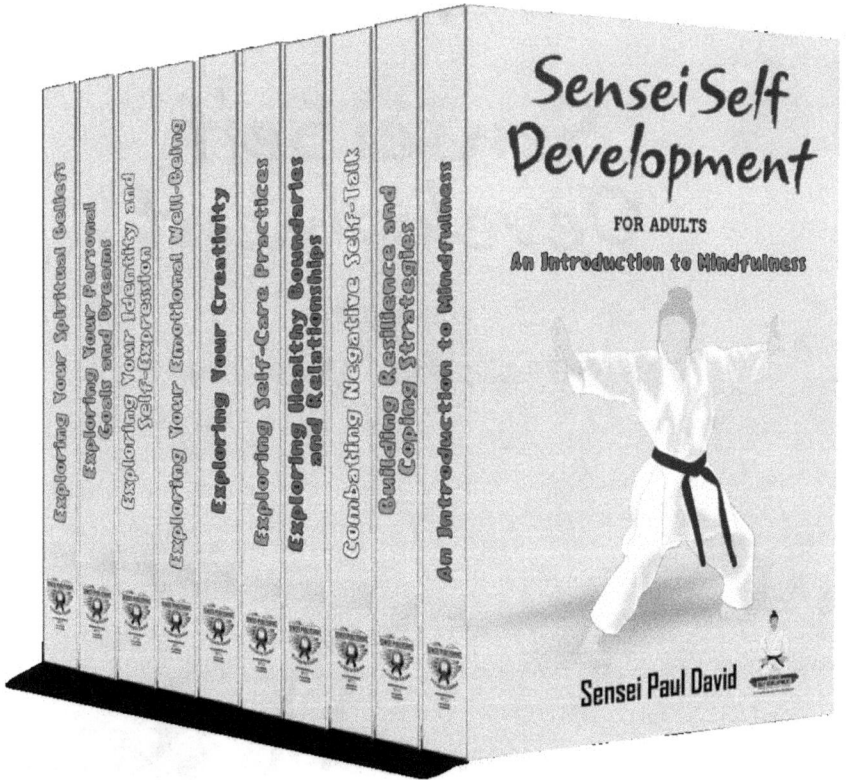

Exploring Your Spiritual Beliefs

Exploring Your Personal Goals and Dreams

Exploring Your Identity and Self-Expression

Exploring Your Emotional Well-Being

Exploring Your Creativity

Exploring Self-Care Practices

Exploring Healthy Boundaries and Relationships

Combatting Negative Self-Talk

Building Resilience and Coping Strategies

An Introduction to Mindfulness

Sensei Self Development

FOR ADULTS

An Introduction to Mindfulness

Sensei Paul David

Dedication

To those who courageously take action towards self-improvement - you are helping to evolve the world for generations to come.

- It's a great day to be alive!

If Found Please Contact:

_____

Reward If Found:

_____

MY COMMITMENT

I, _____
commit to writing This Sensei Self
Development Journal for at least 10 days in a
row, starting: _____

Writing this journal is valuable to me because:

_____

_____

_____

_____

_____

_____

If I finish a minimum of 10 consecutive days of
writing in this journal, I will reward myself by:

_____

_____

_____

_____

_____

_____

If I don't finish 10 days of writing this journal, I will promise to:

_____

_____

_____

_____

_____

I will do the following things to ensure that I write in my Sensei Self Development Journal every day:

_____

_____

_____

_____

_____

Get/Share Your FREE All-Ages Mental Health eBook Now at

www.senseiselfdevelopment.com

Or CLICK HERE

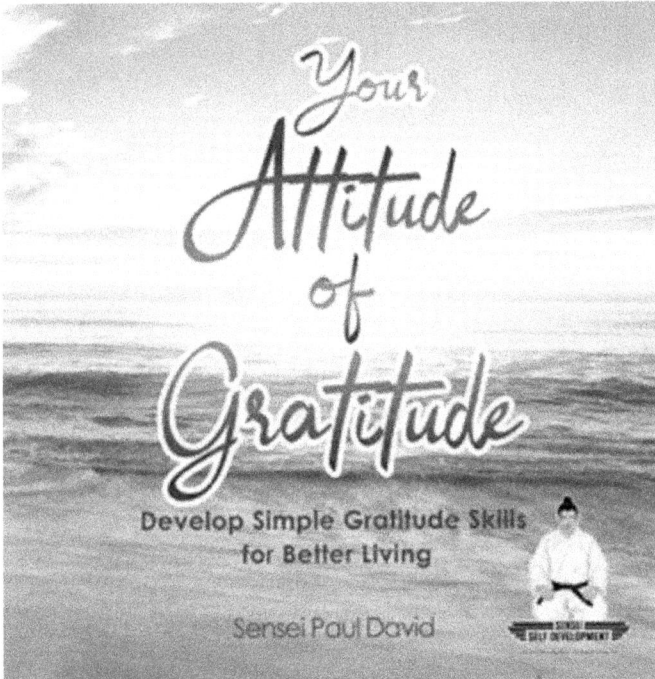

senseiselfdevelopment.com

Check Out Another Book In The
SSD BOOK SERIES:

senseipublishing.com/SSD_SERIES

CLICK HERE

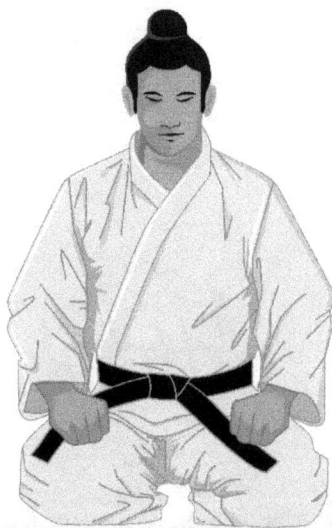

SENSEI
SELF DEVELOPMENT
BOOKS SERIES

senseiselfdevelopment.senseipublishing.com

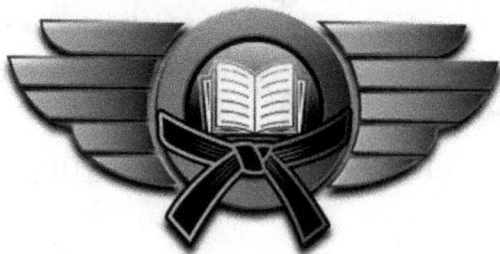

Join Our Publishing Journey!

If you would like to receive FUTURE FREE BOOKS and get to know us better, please click www.senseipublishing.com and join our newsletter by entering your email address in the pop-up box.

Follow Our Blog: senseipauldavid.ca

Follow/Like/Subscribe: Facebook, Instagram, YouTube: @senseipublishing

Scan the QR Code with your phone or tablet

to follow us on social media: Like / Subscribe / Follow

A Message From The Author:
Sensei Paul David

Dear Reader,

Welcome to the world of mental health journaling – a sacred space for self-reflection, growth, and healing. Within these pages, you hold the power to uplift your spirit, invigorate your mind, and nourish your goals.

In a world that often moves at blink-and-you'll-miss-it speed, it's crucial to make time for self-care and self-discovery.

Anxiety, stress, and emotional turbulence may have clouded your mind, making it difficult to find clarity and peace within. But fear not! Together, we will navigate the labyrinth of emotions, and experiences, helping to simplify the path to mental well-being.

This journal is not merely a bunch of blank pages awaiting your words. It is your compassionate companion, offering solace and understanding during your unique journey. Here, you are free to unburden yourself, celebrate small and large victories, and confront the challenges that may still linger.

Remember, the pages you are about to fill are not just a record of your journey but also a testament to your strength, resilience, and indomitable spirit. Cherish this space, invest in yourself, and let your words be an ode to the magnificent journey of becoming whole.

With great respect for your decision to evolve,

Paul

MY CONVICTION

Please circle your answers below

I am DECIDING to be patient with myself and this PROCESS each time I journal toward my improved state of mental well-being

YES   NO

"The present moment is filled with joy and happiness. If you are attentive, you will see it."

Thich Nhat Hanh

Introduction

What does it mean to prioritize? In its essence, as defined by Merriam-Webster, prioritization is the process of arranging tasks in order of importance so that you can deal with the most crucial ones first. This often involves sifting through a variety of tasks and ranking them based on factors such as urgency, importance, and the time required for completion. It's a strategy to help you focus on what will drive the most productivity and accomplishment.

Prioritization can be viewed from two angles:

1. Deciding what to tackle first in a long list of tasks.
2. Managing your daily schedule to ensure you have time for all activities.

Importance of Prioritization

Why prioritize? It's vital for completing everything that needs to be done. By focusing first on tasks that are both important and urgent, you can ensure you have the bandwidth later for less pressing matters. Without prioritization, you risk falling behind schedule, feeling overwhelmed by your to-do list, and ultimately being unproductive.

Think of it like this: Everyone has tasks to accomplish. Many people list these tasks to get a comprehensive overview. However, a list is just the start. The real benefit of prioritization comes when you take those items and decide what needs immediate attention. This approach allows you to get things done efficiently, saving time and energy in the long run. Here are some benefits you can expect to get from prioritization:

- Productivity Gains: Studies show that when people prioritize their tasks, they're more productive. This comes from concentrating on the most impactful tasks first.

- Stress Reduction: Psychological research has found that prioritizing effectively can lead to less stress. When people know what needs to be tackled first, they feel less overwhelmed.

- Better Decision Making: Cognitive studies suggest prioritizing helps in making better decisions. With fewer distractions and a clearer focus, decision-making becomes more straightforward.

- Efficient Time Management: Time management research highlights that prioritizing tasks is key to using time wisely. By focusing on the most important tasks, people avoid wasting time on less critical activities.

- Achieving Goals: Research in goal-setting theory shows that setting priorities helps people reach their goals. Focusing efforts on prioritized tasks leads to more successful outcomes.

- Enhanced Focus and Concentration: Studies on attention and concentration reveal that prioritizing tasks improves focus. People are less distracted and more engaged with their most important tasks.

What to Prioritize

Before we get into how to prioritize, it is important to learn *what to prioritize*. We all know people, maybe you are one of them, who always seem to be working, but the results they get are unsatisfactory. Knowing what to prioritize can help them. I am not talking about the specifics – those only you can determine – but a few general principles to keep in mind.

Keep Track of Your Values to Know What to Prioritize

Staying true to your values is crucial in determining what tasks take precedence in your life. Keeping a consistent track of your values can serve as a compass for prioritizing your daily activities.

Begin by clearly defining your core values. These could range from personal growth, health, and family, to professional development and social responsibility. With these values in mind, assess your tasks and responsibilities. For instance, if personal growth is a key value, prioritize learning new skills or hobbies. If health is a top priority, ensure that exercise and healthy eating are non-negotiable parts of your schedule.

Maintaining awareness of your values helps you sift through tasks and focus on those that enhance your core principles. This alignment not only streamlines your workload but also brings a sense of fulfillment and purpose to your daily routine. It's about making intentional choices that reflect and reinforce what you truly stand for. When your activities are in harmony with your values, you're more likely to find satisfaction and motivation in both your personal and professional endeavors.

Focus on tasks that Will Reduce Your Number of Urgent but Unimportant Tasks

In the hustle of modern life, it's easy to get caught up in endless small tasks, like "chasing cows" instead of building a fence to contain them. You want to avoid repetitive scenarios, such as fixing the same issues repeatedly or giving the same instructions multiple times. To break this cycle, consider strategies like outsourcing, automating repetitive tasks, batching smaller tasks together, eliminating unnecessary tasks, streamlining your workflow, or creating templates for tasks you do often. Identify opportunities where you can invest time once to set up a system that saves time in the long run, like setting up a recurring order for office supplies instead of ordering items individually as needed.

Prioritize Tasks That Are Important, Not Just What's Urgent

Do you ever finish your day feeling like you've tackled all the urgent deadlines but haven't really done anything truly meaningful? This is a common experience. Recent research published in the Journal of Consumer

Research shows that people often prioritize tasks with immediate deadlines over those with less pressing ones, even if the latter are just as easy and offer greater benefits.

It's a natural tendency to want to check off tasks driven by deadlines from our mental list. However, there's a paradox: the tasks that are most significant to us usually don't come with deadlines, unlike many smaller, less important tasks. These important tasks might include:

- Living your values, such as volunteering or spending more time with family.
- Enhancing essential skills, such as improving your understanding of statistics or learning a new language.
- Preventing potential crises, like scheduling yearly medical checkups or developing emergency protocols for your business.

Often, these meaningful tasks get pushed aside as you focus on less important but time-sensitive tasks, like booking a hotel for a conference, sorting through your emails.

Pay Attention to The Big Picture

Staying focused on the big picture can be challenging when you're deeply involved in day-to-day tasks. It's crucial to identify what helps you step back and gain perspective. For me, solo travel, especially flying, provides a literal and figurative high-altitude view that clarifies my path. Spreadsheets are another tool that helps me see the larger picture. While bookkeeping and taxes are not my favorite activities, they force me to look at and optimize my overall financial situation.

Regular breaks are essential too, as they prevent you from getting too absorbed in trivial tasks without realizing it. Another useful practice is catching up with colleagues every few months.

For financial planning, I find reading certain personal finance bloggers periodically helps me stay aligned with my financial goals.

Remember to allocate time after activities that give you a broader view to plan how to apply your insights into concrete actions.

If prioritizing important tasks over urgent ones is difficult, don't be too hard on yourself. The modern world's barrage of deadlines and decisions, coupled with the challenging nature of important tasks, makes this a common struggle. Even as an author who writes about focusing on the big picture, I find it challenging and aim to follow my advice at least 50% of the time. This could be a practical benchmark for you as well.

Prioritize Yourself

There's a common misconception that spending more hours at work equates to being more productive. However, this approach can lead to burnout. It's essential to prioritize self-care.

First, create moments for genuine disconnection from work. This could be as simple as journaling or doodling to clear your mind. Think of it as a daily routine to 'wipe your mind' or perform a 'brain dump', helping to release and not dwell on persistent thoughts or feelings.

Second, it's crucial to learn how to say "no" and set your boundaries. This involves understanding your own limits and ensuring you engage in activities that rejuvenate rather than drain you. It might be challenging, especially early in your career, but being able to turn down requests politely is a skill that enhances your professional and personal relationships.

Third, be intentional about your physical environment at home. Delineate specific areas for work and resist the temptation to blend work with relaxation spaces like your couch or bed.

Finally, have a clear perspective on your career goals and how they fit into the larger picture of your life. Take time to cultivate your interests outside work and remember that your job is just one part of your broader identity. This holistic view helps in maintaining a healthy balance between your professional aspirations and personal well-being.

How to Prioritize

1. Start by Creating a Comprehensive Task List

Before you can prioritize effectively, you need a complete overview of everything you need to accomplish. This step might seem basic, but it's often overlooked in the eagerness to jump into projects. Take the time to write down all the tasks you need to tackle across your various projects. For larger tasks, break them down into smaller subtasks to make them feel more manageable and less daunting.

Once you have your tasks listed, add key details such as:

- The estimated time needed for each task.
- The level of importance or urgency.
- The due date for each task.

Having all your tasks in one place allows you to get a bird's-eye view of your workload, understand the volume of work for better time management, and identify which tasks require immediate attention.

At this stage, don't focus too much on organizing the tasks. The main goal is to gather them all in one location. A good, comprehensive list at the beginning makes it easier to keep everything organized later on.

2. Choose a Suitable Task Prioritization Technique

The way you prioritize tasks will vary based on your job and how you like to work, but there are several widely-used methods that could be effective for you. Let's explore some of these common techniques for task prioritization.

Eisenhower Matrix

One effective method for task prioritization is the Eisenhower Matrix. This technique helps you categorize tasks based on their urgency and importance. It divides tasks into four quadrants:

1. Urgent and Important: These tasks need immediate attention and are crucial for your goals. They're typically deadline-driven or crisis-related.

2. Important but Not Urgent: These tasks are important for long-term success and satisfaction but don't have immediate deadlines. They include activities like planning, relationship building, and personal growth.

3. Urgent but Not Important: These tasks require immediate attention but don't significantly contribute to your long-term goals.

They often involve handling other people's priorities.

4. Neither Urgent nor Important: These are the least important tasks, often distractions or time-wasters, and should be minimized or eliminated.

Fill out the Eisenhower matrix using the task list you have created.

- After categorizing your tasks into the four quadrants, review your 'Urgent and Important' quadrant and start working on these tasks first. These are your top priorities.
- Next, look at the 'Important but Not Urgent' tasks. Set aside dedicated time in your schedule to focus on these. They are crucial for your long-term goals, so planning ahead is key.
- For 'Urgent but Not Important' tasks, see if you can delegate them to someone else.

This way, you can focus on tasks that are more important to your personal and professional growth.

- Regularly reevaluate the tasks in each quadrant, as their urgency and importance can change over time. Something that is not urgent today might become urgent tomorrow.
- Lastly, try to minimize the time spent on tasks that fall under 'Neither Urgent nor Important.' These are typically distractions or low-value activities.

By regularly updating and reviewing your Eisenhower Matrix, you can stay focused on what's most important and manage your time more effectively.

Eat the Frog

"Eat the Frog" is a time management method based on a saying attributed to Mark Twain: "If it's your job to eat a frog, it's best to do it first thing in the morning. And if it's your job to eat two frogs, it's best to eat the biggest one first."

In this approach, the "frog" represents your most challenging or important task of the day – the one you are most likely to procrastinate on. The principle suggests that you should tackle this task first thing in the morning. By doing so, you not only get it out of the way but also gain the momentum and sense of achievement to handle other tasks more effectively throughout the day.

For example, if you have a report to write that you've been putting off, make this your first task of the day. Don't check emails or do smaller, easier tasks first. Jump right into writing the report. By 'eating the frog,' you ensure that your most crucial task is completed, and everything else you do that day will feel easier by comparison.

ABCDE Method

The ABCDE method is a powerful approach for organizing and prioritizing tasks. It involves categorizing tasks into five groups:

- A tasks are the most important. These are your 'must-do' tasks for the day; failing to complete them will have serious consequences. For instance, preparing for a key client meeting or submitting a crucial report. These tasks are your top priorities.
- B tasks are important but not as critical as A tasks. These are 'should do' tasks. Missing them has milder consequences. An example might be responding to important emails. They are next in line after A tasks.
- C tasks are nice to do but not essential. These tasks have no significant consequences if left undone, like organizing your desk. They are lower in priority compared to A and B tasks.
- D tasks are those you can delegate. These might be important but not necessarily requiring your personal attention, such as data entry or scheduling meetings.
- E tasks are tasks you can eliminate. These are low-value activities that don't

contribute to your objectives or personal goals, like browsing the internet aimlessly.

By categorizing tasks using the ABCDE method, you can focus on what is most crucial and make efficient use of your time. This method helps in decluttering your to-do list, ensuring you spend time on tasks that align with your key goals and responsibilities.

The MoSCoW Prioritization Method

The MoSCoW method helps prioritize tasks or project features based on their relative value and urgency, ensuring that the most critical aspects are focused on and completed first. This method is particularly useful in managing complex projects with multiple stakeholders and limited resources.

- M - Must have: These are critical tasks or features that are non-negotiable. Without them, a project or day's work cannot be considered successful. For example, in a software development project, this could be a key feature without which the software won't function.

- S - Should have: These tasks are important but not vital. They should be included if time and resources permit. They are often enhancements that improve the project but aren't essential for launch. For instance, additional features in an app that would enhance user experience but aren't crucial for its basic functioning.

- C - Could have: These are desirable but not necessary tasks. They are typically considered only after 'Must have' and 'Should have' tasks are completed. These could be tasks that add extra value but can be dropped if resources are limited, like additional design elements or minor features.

- W - Won't have (this time): These tasks or features are the lowest priority. They might be nice to have in the future but are not planned for the current project or time frame. They are often the first to be dropped if time or resources become constrained.

2. Schedule Your Tasks Using a Calendar

Every task, no matter how big or small, has a start and an end. Once you've made your task list, assign a start and end date to each item. This practice helps ensure that you keep track of all tasks, especially when new ones emerge or priorities shift.

If you're given a task without specific start or end dates, it's important to ask for this information. Knowing when to start and when it's due helps you plan your schedule effectively and set realistic expectations. You might even want to set your own deadlines a bit earlier to allow for any unforeseen issues or to complete work ahead of time.

Think of your tasks as pieces of a puzzle, with the start and end dates being the edges that define where each piece fits. Your calendar, then, is like the puzzle board where you piece together the overall picture of your work.

Using a calendar tool can help you:

- Balance tasks that require more effort or are higher in priority.
- Ensure you meet all your deadlines.
- Avoid conflicts in scheduling.
- Effectively manage your overall workload.
- Maintain a healthy work-life balance.

When implementing any of the prioritization methods mentioned earlier, or a combination that suits you best, use your calendar as a tool to organize your schedule and manage your time more efficiently. This approach allows you to see how each task fits into your week or month and helps keep everything on track.

Cut Your Big Tasks Into Doable Actions

If you often find yourself setting ambitious goals that you then postpone, try this approach: Think about your goal and then think about a version that's half as extensive. Compare the two and decide which seems more achievable. If the task is still daunting, scale it down further until it feels manageable. You might end up with a goal that's only a quarter or a tenth of your original plan, but it's far more attainable. Starting small gives you the chance to make progress, and you can always expand your efforts once you've begun.

For instance, if your goal is to clean and organize your entire house, start with just one room or even just a closet. If you're aiming to exercise more, instead of an hour-long workout every day, begin with 15-minute sessions a few times a week. This approach makes the tasks feel less overwhelming and helps build momentum towards the larger goal.

Set a Schedule for Important Tasks with Significantly More Time Than Needed

As we mentioned, important tasks like spending time with family, scheduling a yearly doctor's appointment, or learning a skill often fall to the wayside because they are not urgent and we keep postponing them because we are too busy reading emails, helping a colleague, or doing chores. But these tasks are most consequential. They have the potential to cause us the most regret. "I wish I would have learned how to code. I wish I would have spent more time with my family."

To ensure important tasks get done, try scheduling them and allotting more time than you think you'll need. Studies have found that planning when and where to do something significantly increases the likelihood of its completion.

For critical tasks that you've been avoiding for a long time, I recommend a method called "clearing the decks." This involves dedicating an entire day to focus on just one task. I recently applied this strategy to set up a home budgeting software that I have been meaning to use but kept postponing.

Important tasks, especially unfamiliar ones, often have a learning curve and can take an unpredictable amount of time. They might feel awkward and inefficient, which can be a subtle reason for procrastination. In such cases, the "clear the decks" approach, giving yourself an entire day for the task, can be very effective, even if it initially seems like too much time.

To prevent postponing essential personal care, consider setting aside a specific time slot each week during work hours for personal appointments. This can be crucial for addressing medical issues promptly. While you might not use this time slot every week, reserving it for when necessary can ensure you don't neglect important health matters.

Anticipate and Manage Feelings of Anxiety

Handling important tasks often means facing potential worries head-on, as these tasks usually involve thinking about things that could go wrong. This naturally triggers anxiety. Consider tasks like making a will, checking out a health concern, planning for your business's future, thoroughly understanding your insurance policies, or putting together a crisis management plan.

Beyond tasks that explicitly involve worst-case scenarios, even those with potential future benefits can stir up anxiety. For instance, building new friendships, trying something challenging for the first time, asking for what you need, engaging in difficult conversations, owning up to and fixing mistakes, or steadily working on long-term projects that test your self-confidence and resilience are all tasks that can provoke anxiety.

Effectively tackling these significant tasks often requires strong emotional management skills. For example, I find reading works by more accomplished writers beneficial for improving my skills, but it also stirs feelings of envy and self-comparison. Recognizing and naming these emotions is a simple yet effective way to lessen their impact.

Improving your ability to manage thoughts and emotions is crucial, especially for goals that push you out of your psychological comfort zone. Developing robust skills in this area will make you more capable of pursuing challenging but rewarding goals.

Don't Spend Too Much Time on Unimportant Tasks

It's common for trivial tasks to consume more time than they deserve. For instance, you might begin by simply proofreading an employee's report, only to find yourself spending an hour reworking the entire document. To avoid this in the future, consider setting specific limits, like only adding your top three comments on a fundamentally acceptable piece of work, or allocating a fixed time for reviewing and providing feedback.

Developing techniques for faster decision-making can also be beneficial. When faced with a non-critical decision, sometimes it's more efficient to make a swift decision rather than striving for perfection, which can be time-consuming. This approach helps you save valuable time for more important tasks and decisions.

Before We Get Started…

Remember, mindfulness journaling is a personal practice, and these questions are meant to guide and inspire you. Feel free to adapt and modify them to suit your needs and preferences. Explore, reflect, and embrace the opportunity to deepen your self-awareness and cultivate a sense of inner peace.

Date ___ / ___ / ___ : S   M   T   W   Th   F   S

I feel:
(please circle)

because   because   because   because   because
_____   _____   _____   _____   _____
_____   _____   _____   _____   _____

Today I Am Grateful For

1. _____
2. _____
3. _____

What could help transform today into a remarkable day?

Reflective Writing

What values are most important to me and why?

_____

_____

_____

_____

_____

_____

_____

_____

_____

What are some of your core values?

A) Honesty
B) Creativity
C) Wealth
D) Popularity

All Are Correct - Choose The Response You Feel Is Most Important
To Remember

Date ___ / ___ / ___: S M T W Th F S

I feel: (please circle)

:) because _____
:D because _____
^_^ because _____
:(because _____
>:(because _____

Today I Am Grateful For

1. _____
2. _____
3. _____

What could help transform today into a remarkable day?

Reflective Writing

How have my values and priorities changed over time?

_____
_____
_____
_____
_____
_____
_____

Which of the following best describes your top priority?

A) Family
B) Career
C) Travel
D) Social life

All Are Correct - Choose The Response You Feel Is Most Important
To Remember

Date ___ / ___ / ___ : S   M   T   W   Th   F   S

I feel:
(please circle)

because _____ because _____ because _____ because _____ because _____

Today I Am Grateful For

1. _____
2. _____
3. _____

What could help transform today into a remarkable day?

Reflective Writing
What do I want my life to be about?

_____

_____

_____

_____

_____

_____

_____

_____

Which of the following would you consider to be a non-negotiable value?

A) Kindness
B) Fitness
C) Thrill-seeking
D) Material possessions

All Are Correct - Choose The Response You Feel Is Most Important
To Remember

Date ___ / ___ / ___ : S   M   T   W   Th   F   S

I feel:
(please circle)

because   because   because   because   because
_____ _____ _____ _____ _____
_____ _____ _____ _____ _____

Today I Am Grateful For

1. _____
2. _____
3. _____

What could help transform today into a remarkable day?

Reflective Writing

How do I prioritize my goals and ambitions?

_____

_____

_____

_____

_____

_____

_____

_____

What is your main motivation in life?

A) Helping others
B) Achieving success
C) Seeking adventure
D) Accumulating wealth

All Are Correct - Choose The Response You Feel Is Most Important
To Remember

Date ___ / ___ / ___ : S   M   T   W   Th   F   S

I feel:
(please circle)

because   because   because   because   because
_____ _____ _____ _____ _____
_____ _____ _____ _____ _____

Today I Am Grateful For

1. _____
2. _____
3. _____

What could help transform today into a remarkable day?

Reflective Writing

What do I prioritize in my relationships?

_____

_____

_____

_____

_____

_____

_____

_____

What drives your decision-making process?

A) Logic
B) Emotions
C) Passion
D) Practicality

All Are Correct - Choose The Response You Feel Is Most Important
To Remember

Date ___ / ___ / ___ : S M T W Th F S

I feel:
(please circle)

because _____ because _____ because _____ because _____ because _____

Today I Am Grateful For

1. _____
2. _____
3. _____

What could help transform today into a remarkable day?

Reflective Writing

What do I prioritize in my career?

_____

_____

_____

_____

_____

_____

_____

_____

Which of the following is most important to you in a job or career?

A) Job stability
B) Growth opportunities
C) Work-life balance
D) High salary

All Are Correct - Choose The Response You Feel Is Most Important To Remember

Date ___ / ___ / ___: S M T W Th F S

I feel:
(please circle)

because _____ _____ because _____ because _____ because _____ because _____

Today I Am Grateful For

1. _____
2. _____
3. _____

What could help transform today into a remarkable day?

Reflective Writing

What do I prioritize in my leisure time?

_____

_____

_____

_____

_____

_____

_____

_____

How do you prioritize your time?

A) Completing tasks
B) Spending time with loved ones
C) Relaxation and self-care
D) Socializing with friends

All Are Correct - Choose The Response You Feel Is Most Important
To Remember

Date ___ / ___ / ___ : S M T W Th F S

I feel:
(please circle)

because _____ because _____ because _____ because _____ because _____

Today I Am Grateful For

1. _____
2. _____
3. _____

What could help transform today into a remarkable day?

Reflective Writing

How do I balance my values with external demands?

_____

_____

_____

_____

_____

_____

_____

What brings you the most fulfillment in life?

A) Achieving goals
B) Helping others
C) Traveling and experiencing new cultures
D) Material possessions

All Are Correct - Choose The Response You Feel Is Most Important To Remember

Date ___ / ___ / ___ : S   M   T   W   Th   F   S

I feel:
(please circle)

because because because because because
_____ _____ _____ _____ _____
_____ _____ _____ _____ _____

Today I Am Grateful For

1. _____
2. _____
3. _____

What could help transform today into a remarkable day?

Reflective Writing

What do I need to do to stay true to my values?

_____

_____

_____

_____

_____

_____

_____

_____

What do you value most in relationships?

A) Trust
B) Communication
C) Mutual interests
D) Financial stability

All Are Correct - Choose The Response You Feel Is Most Important
To Remember

Date ___ / ___ / ___: S M T W Th F S

I feel:
(please circle)

because   because   because   because   because
_____   _____   _____   _____   _____
_____   _____   _____   _____   _____

Today I Am Grateful For

1. _____
2. _____
3. _____

What could help transform today into a remarkable day?

Reflective Writing

What do I need to do to ensure my values and priorities are aligned?

_____

_____

_____

_____

_____

_____

_____

Which of the following do you consider to be a deal-breaker in a relationship?

A) Infidelity
B) Different political beliefs
C) Lack of ambition
D) Different religious beliefs

All Are Correct - Choose The Response You Feel Is Most Important To Remember

Date ___ / ___ / ___ : S   M   T   W   Th   F   S

I feel:
(please circle)

because _____ because _____ because _____ because _____ because _____

Today I Am Grateful For

1. _____
2. _____
3. _____

What could help transform today into a remarkable day?

Reflective Writing

What steps do I need to take to ensure I stick to my values?

_____

_____

_____

_____

_____

_____

_____

How do you handle conflict?

A) Avoid it at all costs
B) Confront it head-on
C) Seek compromise
D) Try to understand the other person's perspective

All Are Correct - Choose The Response You Feel Is Most Important To Remember

Date ___/___/___: S   M   T   W   Th   F   S

I feel:
(please circle)

because   because   because   because   because
_____   _____   _____   _____   _____
_____   _____   _____   _____   _____

Today I Am Grateful For

1. _____
2. _____
3. _____

What could help transform today into a remarkable day?

Reflective Writing
How can I remain true to my values in difficult times?

_____

_____

_____

_____

_____

_____

_____

_____

What is your top financial priority?

A) Saving for retirement
B) Paying off debt
C) Building wealth
D) Living comfortably in the present

All Are Correct - Choose The Response You Feel Is Most Important
To Remember

Date ___ / ___ / ___ : S   M   T   W   Th   F   S

I feel:
(please circle)

because   because   because   because   because

_____ _____ _____ _____ _____

_____ _____ _____ _____ _____

Today I Am Grateful For

1. _____

2. _____

3. _____

What could help transform today into a remarkable day?

Reflective Writing
How can I ensure my values and priorities are
reflected in my decisions?

_____

_____

_____

_____

_____

_____

_____

_____

What do you value most in a home?

A) Location
B) Size
C) Aesthetics
D) Affordability

All Are Correct - Choose The Response You Feel Is Most Important
To Remember

Date ___ / ___ / ___: S M T W Th F S

I feel:
(please circle)

because because because because because
_____ _____ _____ _____ _____
_____ _____ _____ _____ _____

Today I Am Grateful For

1. _____
2. _____
3. _____

What could help transform today into a remarkable day?

Reflective Writing

What are the potential consequences of not
staying true to my values and priorities?

_____

_____

_____

_____

_____

_____

_____

How important is personal growth to you?

A) Essential
B) Somewhat important
C) Not a priority
D) It depends on the situation

All Are Correct - Choose The Response You Feel Is Most Important
To Remember

Date ___ / ___ / ___ : S M T W Th F S

I feel:
(please circle)

because _____ because _____ because _____ because _____ because _____

Today I Am Grateful For

1. _____
2. _____
3. _____

What could help transform today into a remarkable day?

Reflective Writing

How can I use my values to guide my decisions and actions?

_____

_____

_____

_____

_____

_____

_____

Which of the following best describes your preferred style of communication?

A) Direct and assertive
B) Passive and non-confrontational
C) Compassionate and understanding
D) Humorous and light-hearted

All Are Correct - Choose The Response You Feel Is Most Important To Remember

As we reach the final pages of this journey through "Positive Mindset," I want to extend my heartfelt thanks to you. Your commitment to exploring positivity and its transformative power is not only commendable but a testament to your desire for personal growth and a richer, more fulfilling life experience.

Remember, the journey towards a positive mindset is ongoing and ever-evolving. Each day presents new opportunities to apply these principles, to learn, and to grow. I encourage you to revisit these pages whenever you need a reminder of your incredible potential to foster positivity and resilience in the face of life's challenges.

As we part ways, I leave you with a quote that has been a guiding star in my journey: "The greatest discovery of any generation is that a human can alter his life by altering his attitude."

– William James.

Thank you for allowing me to be a part of your journey. May your path be filled with light, hope, and endless possibilities. Farewell, and may you carry the spirit of positivity with you, today and always.

With gratitude and best wishes,

Sensei Paul David

Reflective Writing

The End

As you close the pages of this mindfulness journal, remember that each word you've written is a step on your journey towards self-awareness and inner peace. Embrace the moments of clarity, the revelations, and even the uncertainties you've encountered along the way. Let this journal be a testament to your growth and a reminder that every day offers a new opportunity to be present, to observe, and to appreciate the simple wonders of life. Carry these lessons forward, and may your path be filled with mindful moments and serene reflections. Until we meet again in these pages, be gentle with yourself and stay anchored in the now.

Mindfulness isn't difficult, we just need to remember to do it.

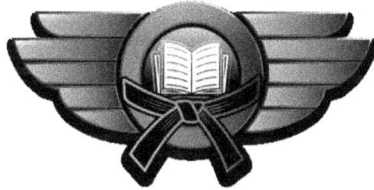

Thank You!

If you found this book helpful, I would be grateful if you would **post an honest review on Amazon** so this book can reach other supportive readers like you!

All you need to do is digitally flip to the back and leave your review. Or visit amazon.com/author/senseipauldavid click the correct book cover and click on the blue link next to the yellow stars that say, "customer reviews."

As always...
It's a great day to be alive!

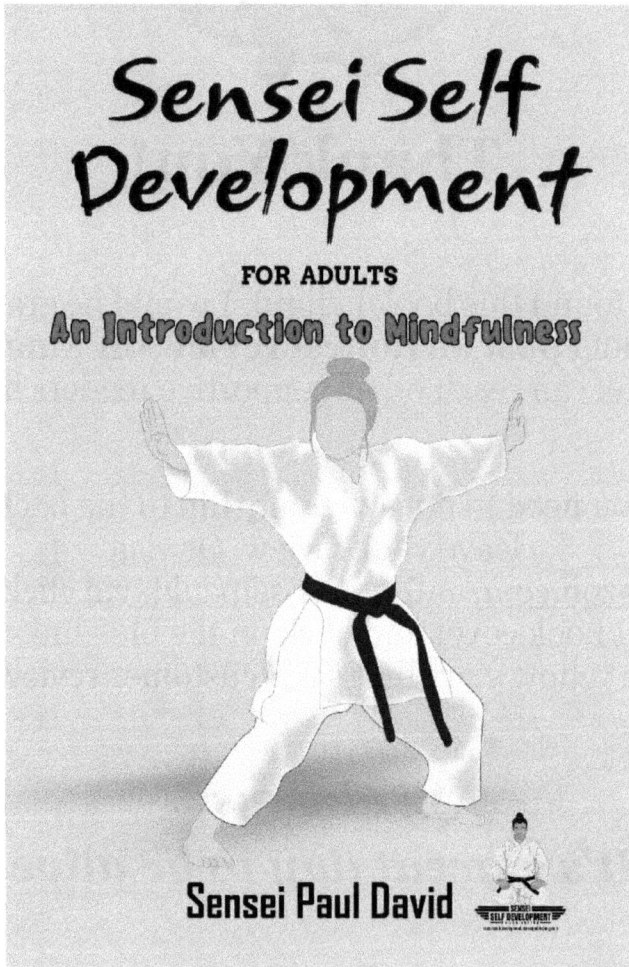

Sensei Self Development

FOR ADULTS

An Introduction to Mindfulness

Sensei Paul David

Check Out The SSD Chronicles Series CLICK HERE

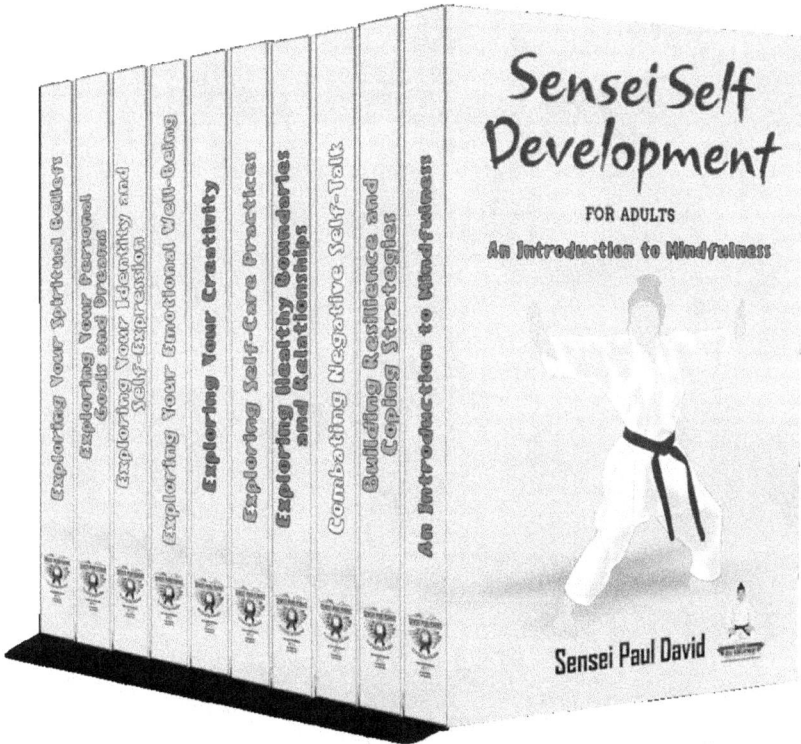

Sensei Self Development

FOR ADULTS

An Introduction to Mindfulness

Sensei Paul David

Exploring Your Spiritual Beliefs

Exploring Your Personal Goals and Dreams

Exploring Your Identity and Self-Expression

Exploring Your Emotional Well-Being

Exploring Your Creativity

Exploring Self-Care Practices

Exploring Healthy Boundaries and Relationships

Combatting Negative Self-Talk

Building Resilience and Coping Strategies

An Introduction to Mindfulness

Get/Share Your FREE All-Ages Mental Health eBook Now at

www.senseiselfdevelopment.com
Or CLICK HERE

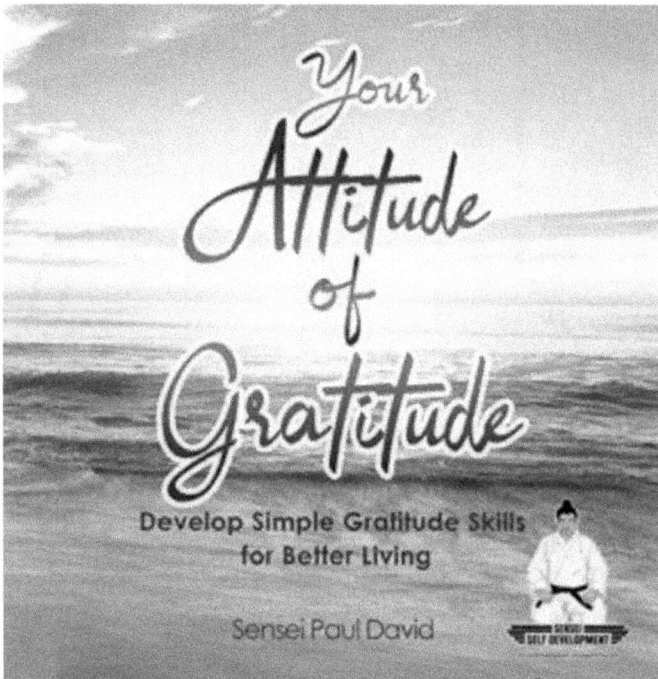

senseiselfdevelopment.com

Click Another Book In The SSD
BOOK SERIES:
senseipublishing.com/SSD_SERIES
CLICK HERE

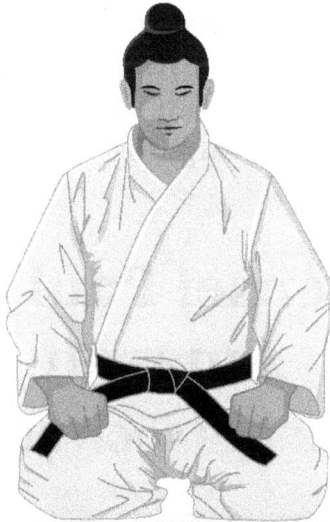

SENSEI
SELF DEVELOPMENT
BOOKS SERIES
senseiselfdevelopment.senseipublishing.com

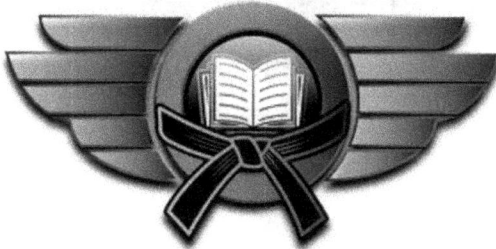

Join Our Publishing Journey!

If you would like to receive FREE BOOKS, please visit **www.senseipublishing.com**. Join our newsletter by entering your email address in the pop-up box

Follow Sensei Paul David on Amazon

CLICK THE LOGO BELOW

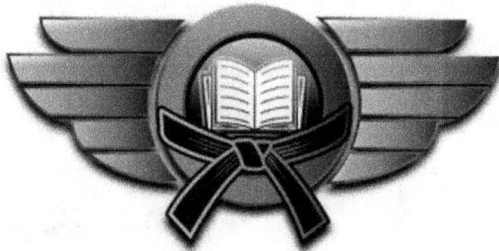

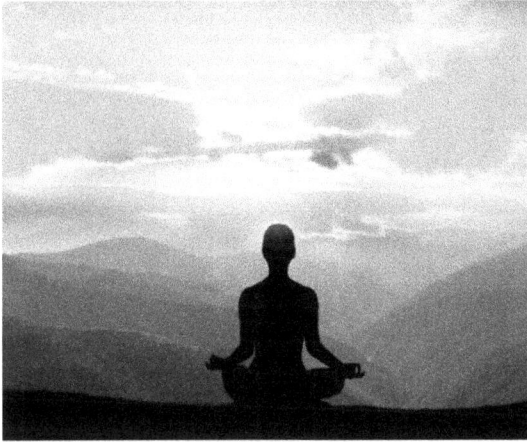

FREE BONUS!!!
Experience Over 25 FREE Engaging Guided Meditations!

Prized Skills & Practices for Adults & Kids. Help Restore Deep-Sleep, Lower Stress, Improve Posture, Navigate Uncertainty & More.

Download the Free Insight Timer App and click the link below:
http://insig.ht/sensei_paul

About Sensei Publishing

Sensei Publishing commits itself to helping people of all ages transform into better versions of themselves by providing high-quality and research-based self-development books with an emphasis on mental health and guided meditations. Sensei Publishing offers well-written e-books, audiobooks, paperbacks and online courses that simplify complicated but practical topics in line with its mission to inspire people towards positive transformation.

It's a great day to be alive!

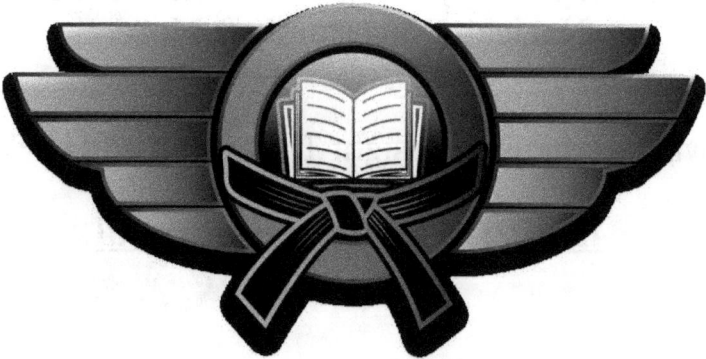

About the Author

I create simple & transformative eBooks & Guided Meditations for Adults & Children proven to help navigate uncertainty, solve niche problems & bring families closer together.

I'm a former finance project manager, private pilot, jiu-jitsu instructor, musician & former University of Toronto Fitness Trainer. I prefer a science-based approach to focus on these & other areas in my life to stay humble & hungry to evolve. I hope you enjoy my work and I'd love to hear your feedback.

- It's a great day to be alive!

Sensei Paul David

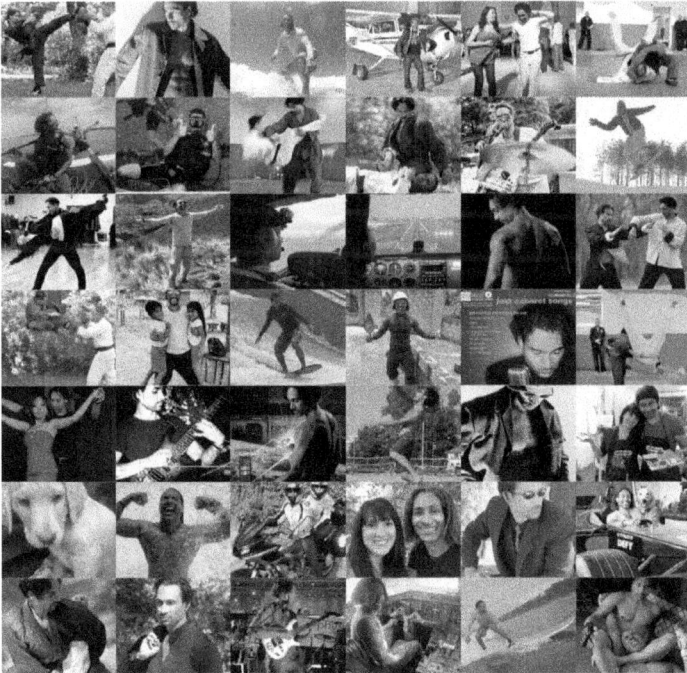

Scan & Follow/Like/Subscribe: Facebook, Instagram, YouTube: @senseipublishing

Scan using your phone/iPad camera for Social Media
Visit us at www.senseipublishing.com and sign up for our
newsletter to learn more about our exciting books and to
experience our FREE Guided Meditations for Kids & Adults.

www.ingramcontent.com/pod-product-compliance
Lightning Source LLC
Chambersburg PA
CBHW071244020426
42333CB00015B/1623